The Anti-Inflammatory Diet: Rescue 911- The Best Foods and Strategies to put out the Flame in your body (Chronic Autoimmune diseases, Multiple sclerosis,Lupus,etc)

I0421397

By Malik Johnson

Table of Contents

Introduction 5

Chapter 1 10

How to Fight the Raging Wildfire Within 10

Chapter 2 17

The Silent Epidemic 17

Chapter 3 26

Solutions to Take the Sizzle out of Searing 26

Foods with a GI Score Lower Than 55......47

Chapter 4 51

Gluten: Inflammation's Deadly Ally 51

Chapter 5 69

Inflammatory Processed Foods: A Packaged
Chemical Fire that Kills 69

Chapter 6 85

Eliminating Food Allergens: 85

Chapter 7..94

Autoimmune Disease and Inflammation: When
your Own Body is Setting You on Fire....................94

Chapter 8 107

Arachidonic Acid: The Omega-6 to Omega-3 Fatty
Acid Imbalance that's Keeping You Sick, Fat &
Inflamed! 107

Chapter 9 125

   Living Paleo: The Ancient Secret that Cures
   Modern Inflammation 125

Chapter 10 153

   An Anti-Inflammatory Lifestyle to Keep the Burn
   Away Forever 153

Recipe Index 168

Other books by author 193

Introduction

A burning sensation wakes you from your deep sleep. You look around in a panic, trying to find a way out but it's too late, up, down, and all around you, everything is engulfed in blazing, red-hot flames. You are on fire.

This is not a figment of the imagination. If you ignore the aches, joint pains and tiredness that are common signs of chronic inflammation, you may be burning your own body down from the inside out.

Inflammation is the raging fire that is at the root of all of the deadly diseases of aging. When this fire spreads deep into your cells it can trigger cancer, when it moves into your heart, it's the cause of cardiac arrest and when it climbs into your brain and burns brightly there, Alzheimer's is the result.

Do you sometimes wake up so tired, you literally have to drag yourself out of bed? Have you become used to that aching feeling in your muscles and bones? Do you find yourself looking in the mirror, wondering why your weight keeps ballooning out of control, no matter how many diet plans you try?

While you go about your day-to-day life, feeling, but paying little attention to these critical signs, you may be the victim of a silent but lethal fire that, if left unchecked, will spread through each and every part of your body, changing you from a strong, active person into a helpless mass of pain.

Let me be very clear: The chronic inflammation that's behind the fatigue, pain and weight gain you've been experiencing is NOT something you can ignore. If you suspect you may be suffering from this condition that is behind everything from obesity to depression, you need to get help right away. The chances that chronic inflammation is the secret cause of your weight and health problems are very high. Nearly 1 out of every 3 Americans can pin the blame for their obesity, illness, anxiety and depression on chronic inflammation. This fire is an epidemic, sweeping through millions of people's lives, destroying everything in its path.

That's why this is NOT another diet book. This is an emergency guide that can help you save your body, your mind and your life NOW, before it's too late! In this book, I'll be sharing with you the frightening truth behind how inflammation can ravage your system and leave you looking and feeling much older and sicker than you should. I'll explain how inflammation can smolder in your body for years causing you to suffer from dozens of different conditions, from digestive disorders to depression, from diabetes to dementia.

You will learn how the common foods you're eating are pouring fuel on inflammation's blazing fire, putting you at risk for autoimmune disease, heart attacks and rapid aging so drastic you can see the deterioration every time you glance at the mirror.

Most importantly, I'll be sharing with you the powerful foods and habits that are your body's best line of defense against inflammation. These foods and habits are the firemen that are ready to rush in and save your body and your life from the terrifying flames that are trying to reduce you to ashes.

These firemen are just waiting to rescue you, so why allow yourself to stay trapped in a burning house? If you're ready to put out the deadly fire and gain health, fitness and happiness RIGHT NOW, you've come to the right place. This book will help you get from the pain, confusion and dissatisfaction of where you are to the joy, vitality and vibrancy of where you want to be. Read on now for the life-saving information you need!

Chapter 1

How to Fight the Raging Wildfire Within

What is inflammation?

Inflammation is your body's natural, protective reaction to an invasion. When your body feels it is being attacked by harmful foreign organisms, it begins a process of attempting to remove the potential danger and healing any damaged tissue. In the right context, inflammation is an incredible and positive mechanism that destroys invaders like bacteria and viruses and heals wounds, keeping you safe and healthy.

To fully understand what inflammation is and how it works, imagine a small fire in the wilderness. This fire is your first line of defense against all of the threats lurking in the darkness, and as long as the flames stay under your control, you can use it to stay alive and well in a hostile environment. But what happens when that small fire that you built for your protection suddenly erupts into a fierce blazing wildfire, spreading faster and wider until you find yourself completely surrounded by a burning wall of flames on every side? That is exactly what happens when your body's small, controlled and protective inflammatory response turns into an immense, insatiable conflagration known as chronic inflammation. If normal inflammation is a safe camp fire, chronic inflammation is a dangerous wildfire that can blaze through every single cell in your body and will stop at nothing until it burns you down!

9-1-1: This is a Health Emergency!

So what can you do to stop this raging, merciless fire inside you? Exactly what you would do in a real-life wildfire situation: *get emergency help right away*. Chronic inflammation is one of the most deadly conditions known to mankind and it is responsible for millions of injuries and illnesses worldwide but you don't have to let yourself become another sad statistic. There are ways to dial 9-1-1 on this out of control fire and get the help you need to save your life. This book will show you how to call up the best and strongest defense team against chronic inflammation and the scorching, searing pain, nerve and tissue damage, organ destruction and death it wants to bring into your life. You'll learn about the top "anti-inflammatory firemen", a group of potent, dynamic and highly effective inflammation fighters that you can access right now to put a stop to the burn immediately. This specially assembled force will beat out the flames, quench the embers and work to cool and heal the damage quickly, for lasting relief that will show you how wonderful and vital life can be, pain-free, weight gain-free and disease-free.

Are you sick and tired of being sick and tired? Have you had enough of crushing exhaustion, weight that keeps spiraling out of control, deep depression and mind-numbing brain fog that leaves you wondering where your sharp thinking went? Are you done with diseases like MS, HS, diabetes, arthritis, lupus and many, many others? And what about those endless doctor's appointments, and the toxic, expensive, often ineffective prescription medications that are keeping you sick and destroying your life-are you done with those too?

If you've had absolutely ENOUGH of being told to suffer in silence and you won't take "we don't know what's wrong with you" for an answer anymore, this book is for you. If you want real answers and solutions to your health, weight and mood problems, you've come to the right place. This emergency guide to regaining your wellbeing and vitality will show you step-by-easy to follow-step, how to gain the strong, fit body, the sharp, quick thinking mind and the happy, youthful and energetic life you were born to have. You will understand not only WHY you're in pain, overweight, anxious and unhappy but also HOW to put a stop to these disorders right away. This is not another diet plan that tells you the same old information that has been keeping people sick and fat, year after year. Those diet books only deal with the *symptoms* of pain, autoimmune disorders and obesity. We're going to be dealing with wiping out the *root cause* of all of these problems.

Those diet books give out ridiculous "advice" that insults your intelligence, like prescribing a high-carb, high-grain, SAD (standard American diet) to help you lose weight and get healthy but this book tells you the truth that doctors and researchers have known for decades: that standard "healthy" diet is probably behind all of your weight gain and illness in the first place!

And most importantly, those diet books are the equivalent of trying to put out a deadly wildfire with a cup of water but this book is the equivalent of calling in a well-trained, well-equipped firefighting force to completely extinguish the flames and rescue you from the pain and suffering you've endured for too long.

Are you ready to save your mind, body and life from the scorching, destructive flames of chronic inflammation? Read on to stop the assault and start the healing today.

Chapter 2

The Silent Epidemic

There is a quiet, invisible killer on the loose and it is making its way into the bodies and lives of millions of people every single day. There is no vaccine that can prevent this epidemic from spreading into your joints, organs and blood, no medication that can turn off the burning, unbearable pain that it unleashes, once it enters. Chemicals can't kill this killer and time can't cool it down. What can you do to make sure that your health and vitality don't become the next victim?

Recognizing the frightening reach and power of this epidemic is the first step in protecting yourself. Doctors and researchers have realized that chronic inflammation is directly linked to almost every single deadly or painful disease on Earth. Think about this: almost every single condition or disease that has "itis" or "osis" at the end of its name is actually an inflammatory disease! But wait, isn't that almost every single disease known to mankind? Exactly! The terrible truth is that inflammation is behind ALL of the modern diseases of our time, especially the so-called diseases of aging.

So what exactly does chronic inflammation do to your body and your life?

Diseases triggered, caused or exacerbated by chronic inflammation include:

- ADD/ADHD
- Allergies
- Alzheimer's disease

- Asthma

- Bursitis

- Cancer

- Celiac disease

- Crohn's disease

- Depression

- Diabetes

- Diverticulitis

- Fibromyaligia

- Gastritis

- Gingivitis

- Heart disease

- HS

- Inflammatory bowel disease

- Laryngitis

- Lupus

- Migraines

- MS

- Neuropathy

- Osteoporosis

- Otitis

- Otitis

- Psoriasis

- Rheumatoid arthritis

- Sinusitis

- Stroke

- Tendonitis

- Thyroiditis

And the truly worrying part is that this list is by no means exhaustive. These are just a *few* of the life-destroying diseases and conditions inflammation can unleash on your body. Now, I know what you're wondering: How do you know that what you're suffering from is really inflammation?

Well, there are medical tests available that can sometimes gauge whether or not you're inflamed. These include a C-reactive protein (CRP) *test* and an ESR (Erythrocyte Sedimentation Rate). These standard tests measure your body's levels of CRP, a protein made by the liver and released into the blood as a signal of inflammation However, while these tests can be helpful in figuring out whether you're chronically inflamed or not, they are far from totally accurate and many times, a false negative can show up, even when a patient is deep in the throes of a fiery inflammation outbreak.

A quick, simple and accurate way to diagnose chronic inflammation is to ask yourself the following question: Do you suffer from one or more of the symptoms below?

Most Common Signs that You Are Inflamed

1. Unexplained or stubborn weight gain

2. Weight gain in your abdominal area

3. Loss of muscle tone

4. Bloating/swelling

5. Gas

6. Food cravings

7. Joint and body aches

8. Headaches

9. Constipation/diarrhoea

10. Fatigue or frequent exhaustion

11. Difficulty getting out of bed in the mornings

12. Difficulty getting through the day

13. Easily distracted

14. Depression

15. Brain fog/ unclear thinking

16. Memory problems

17. Skin rashes

18. Tender gums

19. Mouth sores

20. Fever/ Redness

21. Necrosis.

Note: Necrosis literally means tissue death and is a sign of extremely advanced chronic inflammation! We obviously want to avoid this stage at all costs so everything in this book is geared towards rescuing your health before the damage becomes irreparable.

The Takeaway: If you frequently suffer from one or more of these symptoms, there's a good chance that chronic inflammation is slowly trying to take over your body. But you don't have to let it happen. Even though millions are succumbing to this epidemic of pain and destruction right now, as you read these words, you CAN be the exception. But just like a real-life fire, inflammation can quickly go from being a minor spark to becoming a huge, raging problem, almost in the blink of an eye. You have to take action RIGHT AWAY, if you want to save yourself from years of pain, disease and debilitation. Right now, 7 out of every 10 deaths are attributed to chronic diseases like diabetes, cancer and cardiovascular disease like stroke and heart attacks. What do all of these deadly diseases have in common? That's right. They are all DIRECTLY linked to chronic inflammation. Are you ready to douse the flames of inflammation before they burn out of control? Read on, as we find out how a few things you may be doing every day, are putting your body, your mind and even your entire life in the line of fire and what you can do to put a stop to it.

Chapter 3

Solutions to Take the Sizzle out of Searing Inflammation

Picture this: Every time you wake up in the morning, exhausted and drained, because you had yet another night without enough sleep, you're striking a match and staring a small fire.

Every time you start your day with a syrupy sweet, high –carb breakfast and guzzle down cup after cup of sugar-laden coffee, you're striking another match and starting another small fire.

Every time you skip the stairs and take an elevator or avoid the gym and choose to lie out on the couch, watching TV instead, you're striking another match. That's strike three and those small fires you started are starting to grow larger and more deadly with every bad choice you make. This is how inflammation goes from being a low-level, small fire to an enormous inferno that swallows up everything in its path.

Chronic inflammation NEVER appears out of thin air. There are sure-fire ways that start the inflammatory process and these are the top 7 worst offenders.

The Deadly 7

Dietary Causes of Inflammation

1. Eating a toxic SAD (Standard American Diet) full of sugary, highly processed, highly refined, foods, loaded with chemicals and stuffed with inflammation fueling fats such as trans and saturated fats

2. Consuming gluten

3. Repeatedly exposing yourself to food allergens

4. Arachidonic Acid: The Omega 6 to Omega 3 Fatty Acid Imbalance

Lifestyle Causes of Inflammation

5. Inactivity

6. Letting stress make you sick

7. Sleep loss

Problems AND Solutions

It's important to fully understand all of the causes of inflammation in order to be able to fight them and put out the flames for good. But as I told you in the beginning, this book is not one of those scare-mongering diet plans that try to terrify you into spending your hard-earned time and money on some gimmick. This is not a "problem" book. It's a solutions book. After all, there's no point in discussing problems without providing ways to solve them. I'm all about telling you what's wrong AND giving you practical, real and easy to follow advice to fix it. So when we go into all of the frightening inflammatory damage that everyday habits may be causing your body, rest assured that these vital warnings will be followed with guaranteed ways to beat the back the flames and win the war.

Rest assured, too, that you CAN win this war. Chronic inflammation is a serious, and sadly, sometimes deadly condition but armed with your natural will to live and thrive and the essential steps this book offers you, you can permanently put out those flames and begin living the life you were always meant to have.

Are you ready? Let's get started then!

Because improper eating habits are the leading cause of the modern chronic inflammation epidemic, let's begin with a look at the dietary factors that may be triggering a firestorm of disease in your life right now:

1. SAD: How the Standard American Diet may be destroying your life:

The Standard American Diet (SAD) contributes the lion's share to the mind-boggling pace of rising inflammation cases. It is a diet that is absolutely jam-packed with blood sugar- spiking simple carbohydrates, pounds of tissue-destroying sugar and rivers of irritating, toxic chemicals and additives, all of which combine to ignite every inch of your body. Due to this completely unnatural way of eating, obesity rates in America have skyrocketed from a low 13% in the early 1960's to an astonishingly high 35 % percent recently. When we include the number of adults classified as "overweight", that number swells to a whopping 68%! With 2 out of every 3 adults now being classed as overweight, the simple fact is that we can't afford to allow the Standard American Diet to be the standard any longer!

What Exactly is Wrong with SAD?

Calories: Apart from *what's* being eaten, the problem also lies largely in just *how much* of it is being eaten. Consider this: The average person now consumes 2600 calories a day. Flash back to 1975 and the average caloric intake was only 2100 calories a day. Yes, we see the effects of these extra calories in the form of rapidly rising rates of obesity but the hidden effects of damaging inflammation are less visible, though no less dangerous. With overeating inevitably comes a chronic inflammatory response, so the addition of hundreds of daily calories will definitely have a strong impact on your body's inflammation levels.

The vast majority of the 500 calories added to diets (and waistlines) over the last 4 decades come from carbohydrate sources. The hyperrefined, super sweet and chemical laden foods that you allow into your body on a daily basis don't just sit there, politely waiting to be processed and cleared from your system. They get to work right away, triggering your body's natural inflammatory responses and starting a cell-deep fire, almost as soon as you've swallowed that first mouthful. The worst part is that, with day-to-day bad eating habits, these fires, which would normally run their course and die out, are re-started and refueled. The result is a non-stop, 24 hour burn that shows no mercy to your body's delicate immune balance.

Sugar:

Only 100 years ago, chronic inflammation was a condition mankind did not have to worry about. Today it is the single biggest cause of non-communicable diseases, fueling everything from the huge spike in autoimmune disorders like MS and lupus to the rise of the number one killer, heart disease. What happened? To put it simply: sugar. 100 years ago, people ate only 4 pounds of sugar per year. Nowadays, the average person eats the equivalent of their own bodyweight in sugar a year. That's about 150-200 pounds of sugar a year, per person!

"So, times have changed" you may be thinking. "What's the big deal with eating increased sugar?" Well, there's really only one straight answer. Sugar is a killer. Its effects on the bodies and minds of people are so damaging, so deeply destructive, that it is not a stretch to view sugar as a legal death drug.

Sugar's deleterious properties are best understood when you look at the link between high levels of inflammation and high levels of the sickly sweet substance.

Every time you take consume a sugary snack or take a swig of that super sweet soda, glucose molecules quickly enter your bloodstream. This causes a sudden spike in your blood sugar levels, which signals your pancreas to try to regulate them. Your pancreas responds by releasing a rush of insulin to move glucose molecules out of the blood and into cells which can then employ tem for energy. But when it comes to the 30-60 teaspoons of sugar the average person consumes every day, there's just no way that your body's cells need or can use that much sugar positively. Here's where the problems arise: This over supply of sugar sends your hardworking pancreas into a tailspin, forcing it to gush out rivers of insulin. This excessive flood of insulin and the resulting inability to properly control blood sugar levels set the stage perfectly for a rise in inflammation. Insulin resistance triggers a low level fire in the form of inflammation. This small inflammatory response then triggers even more insulin resistance which triggers (yup, you guessed it!) yet more inflammation.

This terrible cycle continues until what was once a low-level fire burns higher, hotter and more deadly. In fact, it's this exact cycle that triggers type 2 diabetes, so it's no surprise that, when individuals suffering from diabetes are tested, they are often found to be the victims of high-level chronic inflammation as well. While researchers within conventional medicine are still unclear about how inflammation contributes to type 2 diabetes, they admit that studies show a definite link between chronic inflammation and type 2 diabetes development. This link between sugar, inflammation and disease carries further into autoimmune disorders like MS (Multiple Sclerosis), fibromyalgia and others, something we go into in detail later in the book.

High Fructose Corn Syrup and Inflammation: A Liquid Fire Starter

Not all sugar is the same. When it comes to the most highly inflammatory sugar humans are ingesting these days, high fructose corn syrup takes the prize. Research shows just to digest the fructose in High fructose corn syrup, your body must deplete its energy source, ATP. When this happens, it becomes impossible to maintain the impermeability of your intestinal lining. High fructose corn syrup can actually eat holes into your intestinal lining, leaving your body's main defense against inflammatory particles wide open! These dangerous bacteria and undigested food particles are now free to slip past your intestinal wall and straight into your bloodstream where they'll start a body-wide inflammation process that, just like a wildfire, is easy to spark and difficult to put out. This is behind the growing medical consensus that, to avoid inflammation-triggered obesity, diabetes, heart disease, dementia and autoimmune disorders, you've got to douse the flames started by high fructose corn syrup by switching to nourishing, hydrating and natural beverages.

What about Simple Carbs?

There is no doubt that simple carbohydrates like white bread, cakes, cookies and other baked goods made from refined white flour, act on your body's inflammatory response in the same way as refined sugar. This is because your body sees absolutely no difference between the two. White flour is a nutritionally empty, fiber-free substance that is absorbed so quickly (due to its simple structure) that your body's blood sugar levels have no choice but to rise rapidly. This, of course, triggers the same insulin spiking process that sparks the wildfire known as inflammation.

Meet Anti-Inflammation Firefighter # 1: Low –Glycemic Index Foods

In the battle against the raging fires of inflammation, eating low glycemic foods is your body's best chance at beating the burn. Let's take a look at how these foods work to fend off inflammation and what makes them superior to higher glycemic foods.

The Glycemic Index:

In the past, all carbohydrates were simply classified as either complex or simple carbohydrates. This meant that two highly different foods like, for example, baked potato and brown rice were viewed as essentially the same. This ignored the widely differing effects that these two foods have on your body's blood sugar levels. The glycemic index works by allowing you to understand a particular foods impact on your blood glucose, empowering you to make informed choices when choosing the type of carbohydrates to include in your diet.

So what happens to your body when you consume high-glycemic foods? High-glycemic foods like white bread, white rice, potatoes and pasta cause a sharp and sudden increase in your body's blood glucose levels. When this happens, it signals cells within your pancreas to ramp up the release of insulin. This, in turn, leads to an even sharper sugar-crash, as your body reacts to the sudden rise in blood sugar by dropping blood glucose levels to a lower point than they had been before you ate the high-glycemic food. These sudden peaks and pits wreak havoc on your entire system and the high blood glucose levels and ramped up insulin secretion caused by high-glycemic foods leads to a dysfunctional pancreas and irreversible type 2 diabetes. In fact, those who consume high-glycemic foods have a 23% increased risk of developing type 2 diabetes. As we discussed earlier, type 2 diabetes is triggered by and then causes, the kind of insane, out of control inflammation that is the cornerstone of all modern, non-communicable diseases and death. When you eat high-glycemic index foods, you're literally striking a match inside every one of your major organs and waiting for the flames to take over!

 By contrast, when you eat low-glycemic foods, this intense blood glucose spike and rush of insulin secretion don't take place. Your body doesn't have to deal with a panicked pancreas and your blood glucose levels stay even, avoiding the dangerous peaks and pits that high-glycemic foods inflict upon your system. Eating high-glycemic foods has been positively linked to the development of breast and colorectal cancers, stubborn obesity, diseases of the gallbladder, chronic heart disease and even clinical depression.

Have you ever eaten a white flour bagel or a bowl of non-whole grain cereal and felt almost immediately that your face was growing warmer and redder, that your body's responses were slowing down and your thinking was becoming cloudier? These are all symptoms of the rampant inflammation that high-glycemic foods unleash on every cell in your body. Now try to recall feeling the same way after eating a bowl of whole brown rice or a helping of non-starchy vegetables like broccoli or cauliflower. Nothing comes to mind, right? That's because that white flour bagel or bowl of cereal each score a whopping 70 on the glycemic index while the same amount of brown rice only scores 50 and veggies like broccoli and cauliflower only come in at a super-low 15 on the glycemic index!

 It's easy to see why switching those body-bruising high-glycemic foods for whole, natural and healthy low-glycemic foods is like calling in an elite firefighting force to put out your body's inflammation wildfire. Because high-glycemic foods are the common link between this ferocious inflammation and the deadly diseases like cancer and cardiovascular conditions that makeup a silent, lethal epidemic, hanging up on these killer foods is the first step to saving yourself. Calling in low-glycemic foods is the health equivalent of dialing 911 and starting the process of rescuing your body from the health crisis that is sweeping through the world like an unstoppable fire.

Emergency Food Swaps to Make Right Now!

Here's a sample of high-glycemic foods to avoid and low-glycemic wonders to include in your daily meals, to get you started on your chronic inflammation-free lifestyle:

Ditch these Inflammatory Foods:

High-Glycemic Index Foods

- Cornflakes   80
- Bran Flakes 74

- Cheerios 74

- Rice Krispies 82

- White Bread 79

- Bagel 72

- French Baguette 96

- Donuts 76

- Rice Cakes 87

- Breakfast Pastries 93

- Packaged Cake Mix 60-70

- Table Sugar 68

- High Fructose Corn Syrup 73

- Pancake Syrup 69

- Pretzels 81

- Instant Mashed Potatoes 83

- Instant Rice 91

- Instant Oats 83

- Instant Macaroni & Cheese 64

- Pizza 80

- Sodas 68

- Lucozade (glucose drink) 92-93

- Gatorade 78

Switch to these Inflammation Fighters:

<u>**Low –Glycemic Index Foods**</u>

Foods with a GI Score Lower Than 55

- Apple 28

- Grapefruit 25

- <u>Grapes</u> 46-48

- <u>Kiwi Fruit</u> 46

- <u>Mangoes</u> 41

- <u>Oranges</u> 31

- <u>Papayas</u> 56

- <u>Peaches</u> 28

- <u>Pears</u> 33

- <u>Pineapple</u> 51

- <u>Plums</u> 24

- Avocado 0

- Broccoli, raw 0

- Cauliflower, raw 0

- Celery 0

- Kale 2

- Spinach 2

- Bell Peppers 38

- Rice, Long-Grained White 56

- Brown Rice 50

- Quinoa 50

- <u>Black-eyed peas</u> 33-50

- Butter beans 28-36, average 31

- Chick peas (<u>garbanzo beans</u>) 31-36

- Kidney beans 34

- Lentils 18-37

Top Tip: For deliciously nourishing anti-inflammatory recipes featuring low-glycemic foods, check out the recipe index!

The Takeaway: When chronic inflammation rears its ugly head, the main culprits is often a diet loaded with high-glycemic index foods. A quick glance at the lists above clearly shows that these high-glycemic foods are usually instant, pre-packaged and drenched in sugar. As your first step towards a healthy, vital and inflammation free future, switch as many of those lethal high-glycemic items with the inflammation-fighting powerhouses of whole, real, low-glycemic foods. You may find that within just a couple of days, the inflammatory signs and symptoms of flushing, heat, pains and aches begin to clear up without any medication. This is a sure sign that you've already begun to win the battle against chronic inflammation's deadly burn! This is just the beginning. In the next chapter, you'll find out about the toxic inflammatory substances that have secretly been keeping you sick and fat and learn about a powerful anti-inflammation firefighter that can wipe out the flames, instantly!

Chapter 4

Gluten: Inflammation's Deadly Ally

Piercing pain, joints that ache like they've been stabbed with knives and a brain that feels like it's literally burning: These are just some of the reasons why a growing number of people are steering clear of gluten. Studies show that nearly 1 out of every 2 people has some level of sensitivity or intolerance to gluten and even the rarer celiac diseases counts at least 1 out of every 133 people as a sufferer. Research tells us that cases of gluten sensitivity and intolerance have gone up a terrifying 400 percent in the last few decades! It's no wonder that so many people are finding they simply cannot tolerate this health destroying substance. Gluten can light up your body and brain with an excruciating inflammatory fire that attacks every single cell in each vital organ in your body!

But wait, isn't gluten only dangerous for people with celiac disease?

A shocking study that looked at a group of people without celiac disease, who regularly ate gluten, revealed the deadly truth about how serious the gluten threat really is for EVERYBODY: There was a whopping 72 percent increased risk of death in people who ate this toxic substance, even though they didn't have celiac disease! **72 percent**! And the study found that this increased risk of death came mostly from the extremely high levels of inflammation found in the bodies and brains of gluten-eaters.

Some people will try to tell you that, if you don't have full-blown celiac disease, there's no reason to go gluten-free. They'll say that gluten is perfectly harmless and that giving up gluten is just a fashionable new diet. But this study proves them absolutely wrong. The plain fact of the matter is that going gluten-free is not some trendy, fitness fad. It's not an alternative "lifestyle choice". It's quite simply a choice between life and death.

In the fight against the fatal fire of chronic inflammation, the options are clear: Ditch the toxic gluten or let your body go up in a ferocious blaze of flames.

What is Gluten?

To understand what gluten is and why it's so harmful to your body, just take a look at the first three letters in its name: G-L-U. That's right, gluten is a glue-like substance found in wheat and many other related grains. It gets its name from its doughy, hard-to-break down elasticity and is often used in baked goods to stretch out the shelf life of products that should ordinarily be consumed quickly.

In fact, a shocking 80% of all people experience inflammation of the gut after ingesting gluten! When this inflammation occurs, it kindles a raging fire in the gut that burns on and on. As the gut experiences this long term blaze, it begins to become unusually permeable, meaning that the intestinal lining that once protected you from waste, toxins and even food particles becomes open. These strange and harmful substances slip easily past your intestinal wall and into your blood stream, causing a condition known as leaky gut syndrome. Leaky gut syndrome, an often undiagnosed condition, is at the root of so many of today's rapidly rising autoimmune disorders and diseases. With continued inflammation, the cells of the intestinal wall actually begin to die, leaving empty spaces in their place where bacterial substances and pieces of undigested food can rush right into the blood. Your body sees these unusual substances entering the blood stream and identifying them as foreign invaders, it launches a full-scale autoimmune attack against these substances and ultimately, against you.

How can you tell if gluten has made you a victim of leaky gut syndrome? These are the painfully destructive condition's most common signs:

Leaky Gut Syndrome's Tell-Tale Symptoms

1. Digestive distress including an aching, bloated stomach, problems breaking down foods, heartburn, nausea and severe indigestion.

2. Extreme fatigue and exhaustion, even after only minor physical exertion.

3. Aching joints and heaviness

4. Unexplained weight gain and obesity

5. Rampant food allergies. Often, leaky gut sufferers find themselves violently allergic to food they've always tolerated well in the

past and their list of food allergens grows longer by the day

6. Skin disorders including rashes, rosacea, eczema, general redness and psoriasis,

7. An itchy, "dirty blood" sensation that comes from the food particles and bacterial substances invading your blood

8. A deep, burning sensation throughout the body

Leaky gut syndrome is a chronic inflammation of the gut that gluten fuels but it is not the only inflammatory condition that gluten is responsible for. Medical literature tells us that gluten sensitivity can actually cause 55 different painful and destructive diseases! Everything from inflammatory bowel disease, cancer, fatigue, anemia, recurring canker sores to almost all autoimmune diseases including but not limited to multiple sclerosis, lupus, and rheumatoid arthritis. Gluten has also been shown as a causative factor in dozens of psychiatric diseases such as bi-polar disease, schizophrenia, depression and Tourette's syndromes. It's also been shown to be an aggravating factor in a broad range of neurological conditions from migraines, neuropathy, epilepsy and dementia.

In the next section, let's take a look at the frightening way that gluten literally causes the brain to burn itself up!

Leaky Brain Syndrome

While leaky gut syndrome has become fairy well-known in recent years, very few people are aware of its lethal counterpart: leaky brain syndrome. When patients were tested for gluten antibodies, doctors found a shocking surprise: These gluten antibodies were often showing up in patients' cerebrospinal fluid! This worrying finding meant that the blood brain barrier, a valuable, natural "wall" that protects the brain from dangerous substances such as inflammatory or infectious particles, had been comprised by gluten. Gluten acts on your brain in the same way that it acts on the gut, destroying and breaking down the protective lining and allowing life threatening substances to rush in and attack your most precious organ. Symptoms indicating a leaky brain include the classic signs of gluten intolerance, such as:

1. Fatigue

2. A low-grade fever or the sensation of chills

3. Brain fog- inability to concentrate or think clearly

4. Difficulty finding the "right" word or remembering tasks

5. Nerve tremors, especially in the face, such as a trembling eyelid

6. When the condition worsens, facial drooping or loss of normal facial tone

The idea of a "leaking brain" would be terrifying even without the long list of central nervous system damaging diseases and disorders that gluten can then inflict on your body. Gluten, and the leaky brain syndrome it causes, can trigger the following autoimmune conditions:

- Multiple Sclerosis
- Neuropathy
- Facial Palsies
- Nerve Pain Conditions

The inflammation that leaky brain syndrome sets off in the brain may be the main culprit behind the continued rise we're seeing in depression and social anxiety as well as severe psychiatric disorders like bipolar disease and schizophrenia. If gluten ingestion continues, even after inflammatory markers rise, the results can include everything from permanent nerve damage, to the inability to walk, talk and function as a healthy individual. Gluten is the common thread tying all of these life-destroying disorders together so it's no exaggeration to say that going gluten-free is a vital step in the anti-inflammatory diet.

Up to 99% of people with gluten intolerance and sensitivity have no idea what they're suffering from. They often go from doctor to doctor trying to cure the inflammatory weight gain, pain, fatigue and brain fog that gluten causes without realizing that they can cure themselves quickly, easily and without expensive, toxic medications!

If you suspect gluten may be unleashing inflammatory havoc on your body and mind and you're ready to join the millions who've found almost instant relief with a gluten-free diet, keep these simple guidelines in mind as you start the healing process:

Meet Anti-Inflammation Firefighter # 2: The Gluten-Free Diet

Going gluten-free is one of the most important moves you can make in an inflammation emergency. Every time you ingest a piece of gluten-containing food, you're adding fuel to a fire that can engulf your health and happiness. When you cleanse gluten out of your life and switch to anti-inflammatory foods that your body can recognize and break down, you're essentially calling in one of nutrition's most powerful firefighters to quench the burning flames and let your mind and body repair and reset.

Cut out these gluten-containing grains:

- Wheat
- Barley

- Rye

- Spelt

- Oats

- Kamut

- Triticale

- Durum (semolina)

- Einkorn

- Emmer

A quick perusal will reveal wheat and/or gluten as an additive in the ingredients list on the back of many packaged foods. Gluten plays a huge role in the processed food industry, hiding in everything from thickening agents to flavor additives and ingesting these items can secretly sabotage your gluten-free diet. These are the major hidden forms of gluten to watch out for:

- Nondairy creamer
- Packaged seasonings (often contain wheat)
- Natural flavors
- Smoke flavors
- Caramel color and flavoring
- Artificial flavors & colors
- Natural colors
- MSG
- Modified food starch
- Hydrolyzed plant protein
- Hydrolyzed vegetable protein
- Textured vegetable protein
- Maltose
- Hydrogenated starch hydrolysate
- Hydroxypropylated starch
- Vegetable gum

- Vegetable protein

- Food binders

- Soy sauce

- Mayonnaise

- Bouillon cubes

- Chocolate – can contain gluten in flavorings

- Pre-made sauces

- Instant teas & coffees

- Baking powder- can contain gluten

When you first go gluten-free, you may find that your body experiences sudden withdrawal symptoms (we discuss those later.) Give yourself the support you need by getting plenty of pure water and at least 8 hours of sleep a night. It's important to always have satisfying gluten-free meals and snacks on hand to help beat the burn and ward off any cravings so check out the awesome gluten-free recipes in the recipe index, for fulfilling flavors that will make you forget why you ever ate gluten in the first place!

The Takeaway: When the destructive flames of inflammation threaten your health, removing all obvious and hidden sources of gluten can revitalize your mind and body quicker than almost any other anti-inflammation strategy and you may find that your reliance on pain medications quickly disappears as the chronic burn vanishes.

Don't wait for the fire to devour your health and happiness. Make this one simple change: Kick gluten out of your gut, brain and life and rescue yourself from the risk of inflammatory diseases immediately!

Chapter 5

Inflammatory Processed Foods: A Packaged Chemical Fire that Kills

When you enter a grocery store and see row upon row of highly processed foods like cookies, cereals, canned foods and ready meals, what you're really looking at is packaged disease. This is no exaggeration. Dangerous and unnatural additives in processed foods are behind a terrifying group of conditions that are putting the lives of over 35 % of adults in jeopardy! Health-minded people have known for years about the dangerous consequences of eating processed food but now conventional medical research is finally catching up, with studies showing how these "convenient" foods can spark never-ending chronic inflammation in the body.

The truth is, if it comes *in* a can, bag or box, it should probably come with a "flammable" warning label!

Why? Well, we already know that these foods have outrageously high levels of pro-inflammatory sugar, high fructose corn syrup and gluten but they also contain other worrying ingredients like preservatives, emulsifiers, and additives that can stir the body's inflammation response and send you into full-blown autoimmune self-destruction.

The startling effects of these toxic ingredients will leave you wondering if packaged food can really be called food at all:

Emulsifiers: Ever wondered what makes store bought ice cream so smooth and packaged salad dressing so creamy? The answer lies in industrial emulsifiers like carboxymethylcellulose or polysorbate 80. These additives are used to lend packaged food a satisfying consistency and are part of the reason why homemade products often appear entirely different to their store bought counterparts. But according to the latest research, they're also the reason why developed nations are seeing an unprecedented and frightening rise in chronic inflammatory disorders including autoimmune conditions like inflammatory bowel syndrome, lupus, MS, and rheumatoid arthritis. But how can a simple additive cause such large scale problems? Ingesting daily doses of emulsifiers (not difficult to do since they're in everything from breakfast foods to desserts) has been linked to a *doubled* risk of developing serious inflammatory conditions like colitis, insulin resistance and rapid and unexplained weight gain. These are all the hallmarks of metabolic syndrome, a growing epidemic in America. Rather than being one disease itself, metabolic syndrome is a cluster of deadly diseases and bodily dysfunctions, including obesity, abdominal weight gain, depression, infertility, high blood pressure, skyrocketing blood sugar levels and a seriously skewed good to bad cholesterol balance. Emulsifiers work to create this syndrome by eating away at the protective layer of mucus in your gut, allowing inflammation-causing bacteria to flourish and multiply while eradicating "good" anti-inflammatory bacteria. This imbalance ignites an incendiary cycle of inflammation leading to overeating, then obesity leading to even more inflammation. Left unchecked, metabolic syndrome leads directly to the number one cause of death worldwide, cardiovascular disease as well as the 4th leading cause of death worldwide, type 2 diabetes. 50% of all adults are now expected to develop metabolic syndrome at some point in their lives but if you're not willing to stand by and watch your health disintegrate into ashes, taking major anti-inflammatory steps today can mean the difference between life and death. Other inflammation-producing food additives to avoid include:

Aspartame: A no-sugar, zero calorie, alternative to sugar that still satisfies your sweet tooth, what could possibly be wrong with aspartame? To put it bluntly, just about everything under the sun. Long term diet soda drinkers find that when they cut their aspartame habit, they experience a sudden sense of relief: migraines vanish, red, flushed skin returns to normal, their appetites decrease and the dark cloud of depression that's been linked to the toxic sugar substitute seems to disappear into thin air! What could be the secret? A better question to ask might be, why does a substance that's supposed to protect you from the unhealthy effects of sugar cause everything from obesity to painful allergies? The answer is simply, inflammation. Aspartame is perhaps one of the most highly inflammatory substances in the world!

Here's how it sets off a chain of horrifying events in your body. As soon as you consume and metabolize aspartame, it starts to release a lethal, toxic substance called methyl alcohol. By the time this toxin reaches your cells, it transforms itself into well-known killer carcinogen, formaldehyde. With every sip or bite you take, aspartame allows formaldehyde to build up in your body and brain, eventually brining on an onslaught of autoimmune disorder such as fibromyalgia, lupus, chronic fatigue syndrome, depression, and asthma. In fact, aspartame is so highly inflammatory that rheumatoid arthritis sufferers find they experience extreme, unendurable pain after just a tiny dose of this lethal sweetener-a bitter truth to swallow indeed!

MSG: MSG (monosodium glutamate) is a widely used flavor enhancer and anyone who's had the infamous head, jaw and neck aches that follow hard on the heels of consuming foods that contain this substance has experienced, firsthand, its inflammatory powers. After years of insisting on the safety of MSG, conventional research has done a complete about-face and MSG is now known to be one of chronic inflammation's favorite fuels. What exactly does this chemically manipulated "enhancer" do in your body? First, MSG quickly acts on your brain, effectively shutting down its "full" signal and leaving you wanting more and more of MSG-laced foods. This is why MSG use is so prevalent in cheaply produced packaged foods. The drug-like response that MSG induces has nothing to do with the taste of these nutritionally dead meals and everything to do with the way MSG bypasses your brain's natural controls. In the process, MSG actually destroys your brain's hardwiring, causing permanent damage. Next, this excitotoxin triggers inflammation-linked obesity and type 2 diabetes and finally, starts a five alarm fire in your liver, torching your liver's cells and leaving behind burning lesions that can quickly turn into fatal cancers.

If you want to put a stop to the ravages of processed food and take your anti-inflammatory diet to the next level of healing and revitalization, call on this proven firefighter to stamp out the flames and put your vitality back on track:

Meet Anti-inflammation Firefighter #3: The Emergency Inflammation Detox Protocol

When your mind and body are in the line of fire, you need to take real action against the risk of becoming a perpetual victim to chronic inflammation. Whether you've just begun to experience the first pains and aches of inflammation, are already suffering from serious inflammatory autoimmune conditions, or are simply compelled by the facts to prevent inflammation from knocking at your door, this emergency detox protocol is the 1st step in fending off the flames and cooling the damage. Think of this detox as a star member of an elite firefighting team that, along with the other measures you've already begun taking, can quickly and efficiently get your at-risk health to safety.

Step 1: For up to a week before the detox, begin gradually eliminating all sugar, processed foods, high glycemic index foods and gluten sources from your diet and (to reduce temptations) your environment.

Step 2: Begin drinking pure water (preferably from a non-BPA source) as your only beverage. Aim for at least 8 glasses a day. At the same time, limit salt intake to promote proper elimination and reduce bloating.

Step 3: Replace 2 meals per day with your choice of one of the following natural and nourishing, anti-inflammatory juices (You'll find all of the recipes in the recipe index!):

Blood-Purifying Beet and Lemon Juice:
This juice uses the blood cleansing powers of beet and the diuretic effect of lemon to effectively pull out any remnants of your former sugar, simple carb, gluten and additives filled eating habits, setting the stage for the healing to begin.

Inflammation Quenching Spinach and Apple Juice: This juice employs the alpha-linoleic acid (ALA) found in spinach, a substance that reduces a wide range of inflammatory cytokines by over 40% and the quercetin found in apples. Quercetin is an extremely powerful anti-inflammatory, antioxidant and anti-histamine flavonoid, found in high amounts in apples, that is akin to drenching the fire of inflammation in a rush of cooling, healing water.

Burn-Busting Broccoli, Cherry and Blueberry juice: Studies have shown the efficacy of sulforaphane, a substance found in broccoli, in halting inflammatory and destructive enzymes. Broccoli has been found to be particularly helpful in fending off the searing joint pain of rheumatoid arthritis so this is a great choice if you're suffering from similar autoimmune aches. Choose cherries for their ability to soothe chronically inflamed blood vessels and blueberries for their protective and rejuvenating effects on the brain and nervous system. This juice is particularly beneficial for those suffering from migraines induced by additives or leaky brain symptoms brought on by gluten. This juice will douse the heat and help to repair, rebuild and restore.

Step 4: Make your non-juice meal of the day an anti-inflammatory salad such as a shitake mushroom, avocado, and sardine loaded bowl of dark, leafy greens. Shitake mushrooms are packed with the pain and inflammation-fighter ergothioneine, sardines are omega 3 powerhouses (more on omega 3's importance in the battle against inflammation can be found in chapter 6) and dark, leafy greens are full of cytokine-inhibiting ALA.

The Takeaway: Juicing benefits you greatly in the battle against dangerous inflammation. Because the juicing process breaks down vegetables and fruits into their most digestible state, you can easily obtain the potent and life-giving anti-inflammatory compounds and substances found within them, minus the struggle of digesting their often tough cell walls. This is especially useful in cases of leaky gut syndrome, where digestion has been compromised but nutrients are desperately needed.

This detox protocol is an emergency healing measure and should be carried out for no more than 3 consecutive days. Within this period of time, remember to stay hydrated, rest often and circulate all juices, never drinking the same juice more than once a day, in order to avoid allergies associated with repeatedly ingesting the same foods.

Are you ready to feel revitalized and revved up instead of sick, sad and tired? Head to the recipe index at the back of the book to delve into the fresh, mouthwatering juice and meal recipes that will leave you detoxed and flame-free so quickly you'll wish you'd known about this protocol sooner!

In the next chapter, a look at the secret food-foes that you thought were your friends. Also, how to rapidly break free from the cycle of sickness, cravings and sadness that's been gripping your life!

Chapter 6

Eliminating Food Allergens:

Now that you've eliminated sugar, gone for low-glycemic, gluten-free foods and shown those chemical fuels called additives the door, you'll be noticing some amazing changes at this stage. You're migraines have hit the road, those back pins have beat a sudden retreat and your clothes are noticeably looser. Your 3 day emergency detox protocol has given your skin a glow you probably thought it had lost forever. But you're still dealing with other joint pains, with chills, fever, swelling or fatigue. You may be finding it hard to resist certain cravings or to control your emotions. Don't be alarmed. This is all a part of the withdrawal and elimination process that can be difficult but is ultimately leading you on a path of restoration and renewal. If you've successfully implemented the previous firefighters, you're ready for the next essential step in banishing painful inflammation for good.

Let's talk allergies. You may not think you have any but with rapidly rising rates of food intolerances and cases of unknown allergies causing obesity, illness, depression, premature aging and even life-threatening anaphylactic shock & organ failure, it's not a conversation we can afford to skip.

Two simple questions can help to clarify the need for allergen elimination:

Number 1: Do you feel sick, bloated, fatigued, sad or anxious despite trying hard to maintain good eating habits and a positive, healthy lifestyle?

Number 2: If I told you there was a free and easy method to find, pinpoint and eliminate the culprit behind all your wellness woes, would you be interested?

If you answered yes to these two questions, we're ready to get you started on an amazing journey of healing that will see you getting rid of inflammatory deadweight you thought you'd always have to carry and leave you feeling, looking and living better than you ever believed possible! Let's get to it!

Food Allergies: The Inflammatory Link

Unlike the sudden and highly visible signs of an immediate food allergy reaction, delayed food allergies begin by presenting symptoms that are often subtle and hard to distinguish from general fatigue and malaise. However, because these allergies go unrecognized, you're guaranteed to keep consuming the hot button foods, thereby setting yourself up for a catastrophic inflammatory blaze. Stress, antibiotics and sugar are just some of the things that lead to increased intestinal permeability. This permeability allows a sewer-like mix of foreign particles such as bacteria and partially digested food to sweep into your blood. Your immune system goes berserk, beginning to produce major allergies to foods you used to have no problems with. Here's the kicker: The more you eat these food allergens, the higher and hotter your inflammation burns. The worse your inflammation becomes, the more severe your food allergies grow until you find yourself unable to enjoy or even tolerate, a huge variety of foods.

Symptoms of this can include: headaches, weight gain, mood disorders, fluid retention, irritable bowel syndrome, gas, eczema, fatigue and brain fog among others. Many people who don't heed their bodies' warning shots and keep ingesting foods that they're experiencing allergies to end up miserable, sick and weak because they can now only tolerate a poor and unvaried diet! When food allergies can turn nutritional, curative foods into health-killers, it signals that inflammation has reached code red status.

Sadly, many conventional doctors do not give the necessary emphasis to treating these delayed allergies, which they view as of secondary importance to immediate food allergies. It's because of this lack of attention that over 25 million people are suffering in the clutches of debilitating autoimmune disorders. We are now facing what looks like a collective immune system breakdown of unprecedented proportions.

With numbers like these, most people just resign themselves to the idea that they'll inevitably be the next victim. By the very act of picking up this book and seeking answers for your inflammatory issues, you've proved that you're not like most people. You're a fighter, and that's good because beating inflammation takes a fight, but if you're willing to follow this very important step, your odds are better than excellent. In fact, I'm willing to bet you'll win...which leads me to a very special member of your crack team of firefighters:

Meet Anti-inflammation Firefighter #4: Fighting the Flames with Food Allergen Elimination

Do you want to see yourself go from sickly to strong, from sallow to glowing with good health and from being huddled in pain to walking tall, free of inflammation's aches? How about going from bloated and putting on unexplained pounds to lighter, slimmer and less swollen? You can achieve all of this and more in just a few short weeks, with a simple, 2-step, food allergen elimination diet. Here's how it works:

Step 1: Eliminate the following 8 most common food allergens from your diet and your environment:

Soy

Wheat

Nuts

Eggs

Dairy

Corn

Shellfish

Alcohol

Step 2: Record all improvements in your health and after waiting at least 2 weeks, begin adding back the foods, one by one. Carefully note down how you react to each re-added food. The foods that give you the most relief when removed and case the most illness/pain when reintroduced are the ones you should steer clear of, long-term.

The Takeaway: Food allergens can start inflammatory fires that go from spark to sizzle in no time but with the right tools, you can find and eliminate the cause of your suffering. This elimination diet proves that expensive   and toxic pills are not the only or best path to healing. You have the ability to revive your own flagging health by reaching for a guaranteed inflammation firefighter. Try it as soon as you can. You might even feel so great that you decide to do without all the potential allergens altogether!

Chapter 7

Autoimmune Disease and Inflammation: When your Own Body is Setting You on Fire

Your immune system is your body's greatest protector. Every day, it staunchly fights back against millions of health attacks and never stops defending your well-being. Come rain or shine, it stays on the lookout for any potential foreign invaders and as soon as it spots one, it launches a dedicated campaign to intercept the bacteria, virus, parasite or other pathogens that pose a risk to your body and restores you to full health. Your immune system is indeed the most loyal of friends. Until, one day, it becomes your most deadly enemy.

Sometimes, your immune system can become confused and instead of fending off foreign attackers, it leads a destructive, no holds barred fight-against YOU! You never realize the terrifying strength of your own body until that very strength is pitted against you and you find yourself fighting your own immune system, just to stay alive.

Excruciating pain, crushing exhaustion, low-grade inflammatory fever, food and environmental allergies, unstoppable weight gain and intense depression are just some of the hallmarks of an immune system gone rogue. All of these symptoms and many others signal that you've gone from being the beneficiary of your immune system's zealousness to being the victim of autoimmune disease. Over 50 million

Americans now suffer from autoimmune disorders and that number is multiplying rapidly.

Chronic inflammation is the trigger of all autoimmune disease. Autoimmune disease is linked to the overwhelming production of cytokines and chemokines by damaged cells. The more these cytokines and chemokines are produced and amass in your joints and tissue, the more they draw other inflammatory attackers to the areas they're already in. The result is deep pain, heat, swelling, tissue damage and even tissue death. Make no mistake, autoimmune disorders are not merely temporary "malfunctions". They are a sign of a serious system breakdown, which if not treated quickly and properly, can be fatal. With over 80 different types of autoimmune disorders and overlapping symptoms, conventional medicine is often at a loss to provide a clear diagnosis. Some of the most common autoimmune disorders include:

- Rheumatoid arthritis: an inflammation of the joints

- Systemic lupus erythematosus: Inflammation of the joints, skin, kidneys, and other organs

- Multiple Sclerosis: Inflammation in the brain and spinal cord

- Psoriasis: Skin inflammation

- Hashimoto's disease: Thyroid gland inflammation

- Celiac disease: An inflammatory reaction to gluten

Millions of people may be dealing with one or more different autoimmune conditions without even knowing that their everyday aches and pains are attributable to these inflammatory diseases. They may continue to take pain killers or try medications that only serve to treat the symptoms of their condition, without ever finding the root cause of their issues. So how do you know if you're suffering from an autoimmune disease? These are the most common signs to look out for:

- Extreme fatigue
- Muscle aches
- Joint pain
- Weight gain
- Rashes
- Insomnia, shallow sleep

- Gastrointestinal disturbances, IBS

- Sun-sensitivity

- Irritability, anxiety, depression

- Brain fog

- Confusion

- Memory loss

These symptoms are a warning alarm that indicates a systemic inflammation fire is getting ready to take over your body. At this point, it's necessary to seriously assess what may be the secret culprit sparking a potentially life-threatening autoimmune process inside you. Inflammatory autoimmune disorders/diseases can be caused by a bacteria or virus, drugs, or chemical and environmental toxins. While conventional medicine insists that there is no cure for autoimmune diseases once the inflammatory fire has reached a certain stage, holistic practitioners advocate that there are specific methods you can use to douse the inflammation at your condition's root and gradually repair your wounded health. If you're ready to take back control of your body and mind and rescue yourself from the fatal flames of autoimmune disease, the following steps can help you to banish the fire for good:

Step 1: Stop! Drop that Roll!

If you haven't read the chapter on gluten, please make a point of going back and taking an in-depth look at it. Why? Because if you are suffering from an autoimmune condition of any kind, nothing, absolutely **NOTHING** will negatively affect your health more than grains of any kind! Because over 80 5 of your body's immune system is located within your gut, it's vital that you put an immediate stop to ingesting grains that could wind up irritating your immune system even further. Grains have an unusually high supply of phytic acid, lectin and anti-nutrients, all of which have a seriously abrasive effect on your delicately balanced intestinal lining. When you consume these grains (particularly gluten –containing grains), you're essentially allowing them to make holes in your gut's lining, causing leaky gut syndrome. Particles of undigested foods as well opioid –like substances can then freely rush into your bloodstream, leaving your immune system hyper-aggressive ad ready to attack these "foreign invaders." Because of this, your ramped-up immune response goes further than intended, assaulting every part of your body from your joints, to your tissues and organs. This is why grains are believed to be the preferred fuel for the inflammatory fire that triggers autoimmune disorders and why you should always use grain elimination as the first, emergency step in responding to a suspected autoimmune condition.

Eliminate gluten and all grains for at least 60days and see how you feel. You'll likely experience such a drastic improvement in your autoimmune condition that you won't want to continue a high-grain, inflammatory lifestyle.

Step 2: Meet the Ultimate Autoimmune Firefighter: The Autoimmune Diet.

The autoimmune diet is geared specifically towards dealing with the inflammation at the root of autoimmune disease. The main aim of this diet is to remove the "bad" pro-inflammatory toxic foods, replacing them with "good" nutritious, healing foods that your body can use towards its restoration, instead.

Remove:

- All grains
- Packaged, processed foods
- Sugar/high fructose corn syrup/ artificial sweeteners
- Alcohol
- Caffeine

- MSG
- All of the top allergens listed in the food allergen elimination diet

Replace With:

- Real foods including fresh fruits and vegetables
- Anti-inflammatory spices, where tolerated
- Wild-caught seafood and fish
- Grass-fed beef
- High-quality fats such as pure, raw, grass –fed butter, Extra-virgin olive oil, animal fat etc.

Checkout the anti-inflammatory, autoimmune healing recipes in the recipe index!

Actions to take while on the autoimmune diet:

- 8-9 hours of sleep per night, absolutely no less
- Staying well-hydrated to help flush out toxins
- Mild to moderate anti-inflammatory exercise
- Time spent relaxing, in order to boost the diet's potential healing power

The Takeaway: Autoimmune disease has become one of the leading causes for debilitation and death and must be taken seriously. Making this extremely skilled firefighter your choice in combatting autoimmune disorders is a decision you'll never regret. From the first few days onwards, you'll begin to experience amazing benefits from weight loss and pain relief to the end of joint swelling and even renewed vigor and energy. Start today to begin the healing, flame-quenching process and watch in amazement as the autoimmune diet rolls back the damaging effect of autoimmune disease!

Chapter 8

Arachidonic Acid: The Omega-6 to Omega-3 Fatty Acid Imbalance that's Keeping You Sick, Fat & Inflamed!

Have you ever heard that an oil fire is the hardest kind of fire to put out? It's the same when it comes to the fire of inflammation as well. Here's how ingesting the wrong kinds of oils adds fuel to a frightening fire that can rage out of control very quickly!

Picture this: You're serious about protecting your heart from the negative cardiovascular effects of inflammation, so perhaps you've gone to see a conventional nutritionist. According to the advice you received, you make sure that your nutritious, anti-inflammatory diet now includes a good helping of all those "heart-healthy", plant-based oils that nutritionists recommend like sunflower and safflower. Perhaps you've also heard that soy products can offer you 10 times as much inflammation-fighting fatty acids as cow's milk, so you switch out dairy and add soy milk to your meals.

But even after making what appear to be fantastic food choices, something's just not right. You feel increased aches and joint pain, you start to regain the weight you'd lost through the anti-inflammatory diet process or struggle with exhaustion but, like many others, you tell yourself that conventional medicine and nutrition have all the right answers.

But if that's true, then why are you still on fire?

It's time to face an undeniable truth. Conventional medicine has failed millions of inflammation and autoimmune sufferers and conventional nutrition guidelines are only adding to the pain. If you find all your good progress going up in flames after following the usual nutritional guidelines that advocate the use of peanut and safflower oils or tofu and soy dairy, your body is telling you what the nutritionists have failed to.

An excess of arachidonic acid, the result of a skewed ratio of pro- inflammatory omega-6 fatty acids to anti-inflammatory wonders, omega-3 fatty acids, may lie behind your still burning body. The simple fact is that plant-based oils like canola, corn, soybean and others, are big business. These supposedly "healthy" oils are used by major companies in everything from junk food like cakes and cookies to "nutritious foods", like packaged nuts.

Conventional medicine tells you that your body needs the omega-6 fatty acids that are found in these vegetable oils but it never tells you a more important fact: When you consume a large amount of these vegetable oils and soy products, the huge dose of omega-6 fatty acids they contain can strip away most of your truly healthy and precious omega-3 fatty acids! Often, when you eat a normal Western diet, you're pumping your body full of pro-inflammatory omega-6 acids at a ratio of up to 20 parts omega 6 to just 1 part omega-3. The proper, healthy ratio of omega-6 to omega-3 should actually be a well-balanced 1 to 1! So why is an imbalanced omega-

6 to omega-3 ratio important? When this delicate balance is out of whack, omega-6 takes over, bringing about horrific results for your body, including every kind of inflammation-led disease from arthritis to Alzheimer's and cancer to cardiovascular disease.

Here's a breakdown of the difference between omega-6 and omega-3 fatty acids and how omega 6 fatty acids may be the unhealthy fuel behind the intense, chronic inflammation you're experiencing:

What is Omega-3?

Omega-3 is actually a group of polyunsaturated fatty acids, rather than just one fatty acid alone. The main fatty acids of note within the omega-3 grouping are **Docosahexaenoic acid** (DHA),

Eicosapentaenoic acid (EPA) and **Alpha-linoleic acid (ALA)**. These essential fatty acids are the vital anti-inflammatory helpers your body and brain need to ward of the wildfires of inflammation.

Unlike omega-6, these omega-3 fatty acids are found in super-nutritious sources such as fatty ocean fish and energy-replenishing algae such as spirulina. These fatty acids use their fantastic inflammation-beating properties to do everything from preventing Alzheimer's and other forms of dementia, to fending off depression, cancers, eye, heart and nerve problems and have even been linked to increased concentration and cognitive ability. No wonder omega-3s are often referred to as the road to an inflammation-free future.

What is Omega-6?

Like omega-3, omega -6 is a group of polyunsaturated fatty acids, rather than just one fatty acid alone. The main fatty acids of note within the omega-6 grouping are linoleic acid (LA) and arachidonic acid (AA). **Linoleic acid (LA)** is an essential fatty acid that must be obtained through your diet. However, because of an over-abundance of so-called "natural" vegetable oils, most people today receive an excessive and harmful amount of linoleic acid. In fact, people now eat nearly 75 *whole pounds* of these treacherous vegetable oils!

Arachidonic acid (AA) is the second member of this grouping and presents a serious threat to your health. It's also derived mainly from vegetable oils and unfermented soy products and can create eicosanoids, substances that produce inflammation. Because arachidonic acid is responsible for exposing your body to the inflammation-making eicosanoids and because an excess of arachidonic can wipe out the benefits of valuable anti-inflammatory omega-3, it's absolutely vital to limit omega-6 in your diet to prevent the long-term boil of chronic inflammation.

Another consideration that can help you decide to get rid of vegetable oils for good is the way these oils are produced. Unlike the anti-inflammatory and soothing coconut, olive and avocado oils, the health-destroying omega-6 vegetable oils are not cold pressed. Rather, they undergo a completely unnatural extraction process that involves heating their sources at intensely high temperatures, causing the oils to instantly become rancid. Then these oils are mixed with petroleum products, treated with harsh acids, deodorized and processed with industrial chemicals before winding up at your table as bizarre, barely edible products that are basically bottled inflammation.

So what should your reaction be to all of the "nutritional nonsense" that advocates the use of these oils as staples in your diet? A firm NO WAY will guarantee that your body won't be the next victim to fall into the trap of becoming less healthy and more inflamed because of these supposedly "healthy" substances.

Meet Anti-Inflammation Firefighter # 5: Natural Cooking Fats and Oils that Can Defeat Inflammation's Burn

Reject these lethal, pro-inflammatory oils:

- Cottonseed oil
- Canola oil
- Safflower oil
- Soybean oil
- Sunflower oil
- Corn oil
- Peanut oil

Replace with these anti-inflammatory miracle oils:

Extra-virgin olive oil: This restorative oil boasts anti-inflammatory effects similar to medications such as Ibuprofen, without any of the negative properties. EVOO works naturally to repair the damage done by chronic inflammatory conditions in areas such as the brain, the heart, the skin and the nervous system!

Coconut oil: Chockfull of pain-killing lauric acid, cold pressed coconut oil may just be one of nature's most anti-inflammatory foods. Studies show that coconut oil's antioxidants act to reduce swelling, redness, pain and other signs of chronic inflammation so use this fantastic firefighter in everything from breakfast foods to smoothies and watch the flames vanish.

Avocado oil: Less well-known than the two oils above, cold pressed avocado oil still packs an amazing punch when it comes to reducing inflammation. This golden oil is loaded with anti-inflammatory substances ranging from monounsaturated fatty acids (the truly heart healthy option) to carotenoids, lutein and vitamin E, all of which make this oil the best kept secret firefighter on your inflammation-eradicating team. As an added bonus, this oil (which has similar cooking stability to olive oil) is also a known belly fat-banisher, meaning that you can benefit from the oil's properties and the anti-inflammation boost of losing dangerous abdominal fat!

A Top Tip on Using Cooking Oils: Although these oils are excellent additions to your anti-inflammation diet, keep in mind that the less you cook any oil or fat, the better your inflammation-fighting outcomes will be. Go for fresh, whole recipes like tossed salads, using these oils as the perfect dressings and when cooking, apply the oil you're using at the very end of the cooking process, subjecting it to the bare minimum of heat. This way, you'll prevent the oil from going rancid and protect your body from any additional inflammation.

Meet Anti-Inflammation Firefighter #6: Anti-Inflammatory Oils for Supplementation:

The following oils can give your efforts a boost and offer your body fast anti-inflammatory results if you take care to ensure proper storage and dosage.

Flaxseed Oil: Flaxseed oil has long been considered the king of seed oils for its excellent combination of omega-3 fatty acids (1 teaspoon alone contains twice the daily omega-3 found in the average diet!) hormone-balancing lignans and plant estrogens (phytoestrogens). Flaxseed oil is frequently prescribed as an alternative health measure in cases of lupus inflammation and its joint-soothing and neuropathy-healing properties are well-documented. However, it's important to remember that flaxseed does contain omega-6 fatty acids along with its abundant supply of omega-3 fatty acids so caution in dosing is required to maintain the optimal omega-3 to omega-6 balance for health.

Black Currant Seed Oil: One of the most anti-inflammatory oils available, black currant seed oil has been found to be useful in reducing the pain, swelling and stiffness associated with rheumatoid arthritis as well as in alleviating the dry-eye conditions in other inflammation based diseases. While black currant seed oil can form a part of a healthy anti-inflammatory diet, it's very important not to take large doses of this supplement as adverse effects include headaches, intestinal problems and even a strong immune reaction to the oil. Additionally, although this oil contains an almost balanced amount of omega-3 to omega-6 fatty acids, taking it in larger doses may contribute to a disproportionally high amount of omega-6 circulating in the body. To avoid this pro-inflammatory effect and reap the benefits of this supplement, always choose a cold pressed oil and keep daily doses below 1 gram for adults and well below 500 mg for children.

Krill Oil: Studies point to krill oil as being up to 48 times more potent than fish oil, allowing for

---

lower dosage with better results. Krill oil also contains phospholipids, meaning that the omega-3 in the oil is already in a form that your body can use right away.

The bioavailability of krill oil also means it can easily cross the blood brain barrier (BBB), allowing it to effectively ease the brain-inflammation that causes everything from depression to dementia. Making krill oil a part of your anti-inflammatory diet is one of the simplest and best ways to safeguard your brain from the ravages of chronic inflammation.

A Top Tip on Storing Oils: The way you store your oils is just as vital a concern as which oils you use, when trying to fight inflammation. Make sure that all oils are stored in cool area, away from heat sources to avoid potentially inflammation-causing rancidity.

If you start making these changes in the type of oils you consume and the ways in which you use them, you'll start to reap the full rewards of all your hard work in carrying out the previous anti-inflammatory steps in other chapters.

In the next chapter, you'll be introduced to the most highly-specialized inflammation firefighter of all and learn the simple, effective secrets to a slim, ultra-fit body, a sharp, focused mind and an endless fountain of energy that will make you feel like you've suddenly turned back the clock. Are you ready to change the way you look, the way you feel, the way you think, live and even sleep? Well, then what are you waiting for? The solutions to banish chronic inflammation and take your repair, revitalization and healing to the ultimate next level, are only a page away. See you there!

Chapter 9

Living Paleo: The Ancient Secret that Cures Modern Inflammation

Congratulations! If you've followed the 6 previous steps, you've effectively set the stage for the most important healing step you will ever take in your life. What you're about to learn now will be like calling the most advanced fireman from an elite force to put out the fire that's been blazing a destructive path through your body.

The firefighter you're about to access is the only one that is fully equipped with all of the training, techniques and skills needed to completely WIPE out the chronic inflammation wildfire inside you and take you from being a victim of pain, unhealthy, unhappy and always tired, to being the physically fit, pain-free, positive, and vibrant individual you were **BORN** to be.

That's because this top-level firefighter will harness all of the superior healing powers of the best anti-inflammatory methods to give you:

Health: The amazing techniques used by this firefighter put an immediate stop to the inflammation raging through every cell in your body. The results are immediate relief and healing that will allow you total freedom from the world's most deadly diseases including: Heart disease, strokes, diabetes, obesity, cancer, autoimmune disorders and even neurological diseases such as Alzheimer's, Parkinson's and multiple sclerosis!

Weight Loss: Watch in amazement as your body begins to drop years of stubborn inflammatory fat easily and naturally, almost without trying. Many people who call in this firefighter to deal with the aches and pains of chronic inflammation are pleasantly surprised with the bonus of intuitive weight loss and toning that comes along with the elimination of inflammation. Abdominal weight, which is linked to deep systemic inflammation, literally vanishes when this firefighter gets to work.

Rejuvenated Skin: Inflammation can burn you from the inside out, giving you old, tired and burnt-out looking skin. While dousing the flames within you, this powerful firefighter will also effectively turn back the clock on the signs of ageing: Within weeks, you'll be surprised at how wrinkles seem to disappear and deep lines re-fill themselves. With the destructive inflammatory process stamped out, your skin will be able to naturally rebuild its own collagen structure, giving you results that no expensive lotions or serums could ever achieve!

A Sharp Mind: One of the saddest parts of suffering from chronic inflammation is the loss of optimal brain functioning as inflammatory cytokines and a compromised blood brain barrier attack your most important organ day and night. With this firefighter, inflammatory brain problems like brain fog, memory loss, slowed-thinking and reaction quickly begin to reverse. You'll find your mind set free of all the burdens and revitalized, allowing you to succeed and thrive as you'd always hoped.

Improved Mood and Sleep: The same inflammatory compounds that compromise your brain's ability to think and reason also launch full-scale assaults on its ability to stabilize your mood. Chronic inflammation and clinical depression go hand-in-hand so if you're worried that the burning wildfire inside you is causing you to lose the enjoyment and pleasure you used to have in life, call on this firefighter to put out the burn and let the healing begin! You'll find that as treatment progresses, you feel not only physically lighter but emotionally free of all the deadweight of anxiety and sadness that inflammation has been saddling you with. This firefighter harnesses natural tools to give you deep, restorative and truly healing sleep that will help your body to repair every organ, bone and muscle.

And so much more!

I'm sure that by now, you've heard more than enough and you're 100% ready to find out what to do next to access this total healing. If this was another diet book, this would be the part where you're told to buy a certain branded weight loss system or invest in an expensive type of supplement. But here's what you need to know: The firefighter I'm about to introduce you to works for free! That's right-free! No fancy equipment or costly pills could ever offer you the healing that you require. This firefighter's methods are 100% natural and can be accessed by anyone, anywhere, to stamp out the dangerous chronic fire and replace it with rejuvenation.

Here's the one and only catch: it takes willpower.

All you need to do to start feeling immediate relief and seeing immediate results is DECIDE that you've had enough of the painful, debilitating and destructive effects of inflammation. And if you've gotten this far, there's no reason at all why you can't go all the way and reap the rewards of an inflammation-free life. So if you're ready to make that change and watch your body, mind and life totally transform, here goes:

Meet the Ultimate Inflammation Firefighter#7: The Paleo Diet-Eating Wild, Living Pain and Disease-Free

You may have seen the paleo diet mentioned on blogs, fitness websites and even popular TV health shows. If you haven't tried it yet, or aren't even sure what "paleo" means, you may be wondering what all the fuss is about? Isn't it just another fad-diet, that's sure to quickly fade away and be replaced with a new fitness trend of the moment?

The answer is that Paleo (short for Paleolithic) is actually not a new fitness fashion but refers to an ancient, time-honored and authentic way of eating, exercising and living that works with your body's natural rhythms, processes and cycles to leave you in the best shape of your life. Paleo encompasses an entire lifestyle and that's exactly what makes it completely different from any of the passing diet crazes out there.

You don't just EAT paleo; you have to BE paleo in order to see the amazing anti-inflammatory, anti-obesity and even anti-illness results that this way of life offers you.

Here's what you need to know:

Get to Know Yourself:

You are a hunter-gatherer. You may wear modern clothing, use a car to get around and easily access meals by choosing from a restaurant menu instead of stalking your prey through a forest but those are just minor details. Despite all of the changes that a modern lifestyle has brought to mankind, it still has not and cannot change the way your body intrinsically functions.

Your ancestors were active, healthy and strong people who lived lives that were free from the health-destroying effects of chronic inflammation. They weren't burning from the inside out with obesity, fatigue or heart disease. Their immune systems didn't launch friendly-fire assaults against them with diseases like diabetes, rheumatoid arthritis, dementia, depression, lupus, HS or multiple sclerosis. They moved easily, maintained fit and toned physiques full of powerful muscle and free of inflammatory fat, had very few digestive problems and even fewer allergies. They relished their sleep, lived by the natural cycles of day and night and enjoyed the close bond of family and kinship. In short, they were the embodiment of what we mean when we talk about health today. That's all well and good, you may be thinking, but we're completely different these days. And you're right, nothing could be further removed from that life of vitality and vigor than the state that the average human adult is in now:

We are a world on fire. Chronic inflammation has gotten hold of millions upon millions of people, wreaking havoc on our collective health and starting low-grade fires that are never put out and end up developing into unstoppable wildfires that burn endlessly until lives are lost to terrifying conditions like diabetes, obesity, cardiovascular disease and dementia. Weight loss has become one of the most talked about subjects in our lives but also one of the most seemingly impossible to achieve goals.

More people are on cholesterol lowering drugs now than at any other time in history and guess what? More people are dying of heart disease than ever before, too! People are stuck on the high-inflammation ride from hell, taking expensive prescriptive medications to put out one inflammatory fire that only end up starting another, even more inflammatory fire in a different area of the body The result is pain, exploding levels of weight gain and disease as well as an unprecedented rise in depression. It's all true, that's the way things are now.

But that's not the way they have to be.

If everyone, everywhere, lived in the same inflammatory nightmare, we would have no choice but to accept that life today HAS to include pain, disease and early death. But they don't. Even now, thousands of years later there are people living in many areas of the world, who have pain and inflammation-free minds and bodies and these people show us that even though the times have changed, what our bodies need and how they work, have essentially stayed the same. Examples of the amazing power of ancient, intuitive eating and living habits can be seen in the populations found in so-called "Blue Zones". In these areas,, people live healthy, inflammation-free and fulfilled lives and reach the age of 100 years old at times the average rate!

So what's their secret? Well, in Okinawa for instance, the inhabitants enjoy one of the highest rates of longevity in the world, beating out even their fellow Japanese (Japan has the highest rate of longevity in the world!) by consuming fewer total calories, making fatty fish omega-3s a major part of their diets and living in close-knit families. In another Blue Zone, the Sardinians of Italy also boast exceptional longevity and though they live in a completely different continent, their lifestyles are startlingly similar to the Okinawans of Japan. For example, the Sardinians also eat a diet that is filling but nowhere near as calorie dense as the average Western diet. They also ingest a great deal of omega-3fatty acids and have close family and friendship bonds that have been shown to have anti-inflammatory effects. Both of these Blue Zone people (and all Blue Zone people in general) participate in a large amount of movement. This is not necessarily "exercise" in the way that we think of it today. They don't "hit the gym", instead getting plenty of natural activity such as long walks and hard work that keep them healthy without setting off the inflammatory alarm bells that the kind of over-done exercise routines we've adopted often do. These people are a perfect example of living as our ancestors did and their longevity alone is proof of the intensely anti-inflammatory properties of such a lifestyle. Chronic inflammation is at the root of all deadly non-communicable diseases and is particularly to blame for rapid ageing and pre-mature death so the fact that these people reach regularly reach 100 years of age shows that their way of life can vanquish chronic inflammation's powerful fires!

That's what Paleo is about. Going back to a healthy, real and authentic way of eating and living that works like no other artificial "diet" ever can, to give you amazing pain, inflammation, disease and weight gain-busting results that you can start to really see in as little as 7 days. In fact, I'm offering you a challenge. Read the following guidelines and explanations on going Paleo and implement them in your life for just 1 week and I guarantee you that no matter how severe your inflammatory pain or how stubborn your inflammatory weight gain, you will see real results.

In fact, I'm willing to bet that you'll be hooked. Not because Paleo is easy. It's not. It may be the best and most natural thing you can do for your body but trust me, after years of being hooked on unnatural foods, chemical-loaded beverages and substances and way of life that has removed you from nature, your body will want to fight the amazing nourishing changes you're forcing it to make. That's 100% normal. You may get cravings and headaches and maybe around day 3, you might even consider quitting, but if you stick with it for 7 days, you'll definitely get a taste of the kind of pain relief, weight loss and inflammation reduction that NO other eating plan, diet or medication can give you. This is why Paleo is the very best firefighter on the anti-inflammation team, because it's the only one that has what your body truly needs, to put out the burn for good. Up for the challenge? Great! This will be the best health decision you ever make.

What is Paleo and What isn't?

When we refer to something as being Paleo, it basically means that that food, drink, exercise method or lifestyle matches with the inflammation-free habits of ancient people. If something is referred to as Paleo, it's good for your body and mind and great for reducing inflammation.

The opposite is also true: If something is referred to as not Paleo, steer clear of it during your challenge. It means that whatever that something is, it's definitely not good for your body and mind and can further ignite inflammation instead of putting it out.

PALEO

Vegetables

- You can eat all the vegetables you want, no limits! They're excellent sources of nutrition

and anti-inflammatory powerhouses. The
bonus is that you simply can't gain weight
from them, no matter how many helpings of
spinach or cauliflower you enjoy!

- Limit your consumption of starchy vegetables
in the evenings or generally, if you want to
produce the best anti-inflammatory and
weight loss effects.

Fruits

- You can eat as much fruit as you want but
choose low-glycemic fruits when eating in the
evenings

Meats

- All natural meats from grass-fed, pastured animals as well as free-range eggs are Paleo and you can eat unrestricted amounts of these.

- Avoid grain-fed meat and milk as well as eggs from non-free range chickens (Grain-fed and caged animals produce food products with high levels of pro-inflammatory omega-6!).

Fish & Seafood

- Eat wild–caught fish and seafood in abundance

Nuts & Seed

- Eat Walnuts

- Cashews

- Almonds

- Hazelnuts

- Pecans

- Pumpkin seeds

Dairy

- There is some controversy about whether dairy can be considered Paleo or not. The best advice is to pay attention to how you feel after consuming dairy and decide for yourself based on that.

- Full-fat, raw dairy from grass-fed animals is acceptable as long as you do not have any adverse reaction to dairy.

Fats

- Extra virgin olive oil

- Coconut oil/milk

- Avocado oil

- Flaxseed oil

- Hazelnut oil

- Extra Virgin Olive oil

- Macadamia oil

- Walnut oil

- Hazelnut oil

- Unrefined Red Palm oil

- Full-fat butter

- Ghee

- Tallow

- Lard

Beverages

- Filtered or spring water

- Herbal teas

- Paleo smoothies

- Green juices

These are just some of the fresh, delicious choices you have when eating Paleo. When making meal decisions, remember to ask yourself if the food would have been available to your ancient ancestors. When it comes to vital, real, whole fruits, vegetables and meats, the answer is yes and those foods will heal your body and quench the inflammation within you!

The following foods are to be avoided at all costs, because they fuel the chronic inflammatory fires that are destroying your health, making you gain weight, keeping you cloudy–headed and off kilter.

<u>NOT PALEO</u>

- Refined sugar

- Salt

- All grains

- Legumes

- Corn

- Soy

- Processed oils (these pass through several chemical processes and cannot be considered natural.)

- Processed foods

- Alcohol is not considered Paleo

Now, this may seem like a large amount of food to exclude from your diet but the truth is that once you start eating Paleo, you'll find that you have endless and delicious options that you can enjoy without fearing health problems or weight gain.

Now I Understand Paleo, What's Primal?

Primal eating is similar to Paleo in that it's based on ancient, ancestral eating patterns but unlike Paleo, Primal eating allows for:

- More consumption of saturated fats

- Free consumption of eggs

- An emphasis on consuming nutrient-rich organ meats

It's important to strike the right balance for your body but in general, including the foods allowed in Primal eating greatly contributes to the anti-inflammatory and healing effects of this lifestyle. Now, let's take a look at how Paleo eating and living is the single most powerful inflammation firefighter you can call in. In these first 7 days:

- You'll start to see immediate weight loss (particularly abdominal weight loss), even without additional exercise. This is, in part, due to the removal of refined sugar from your diet. With sugar gone, your body goes into healing mode and all of the

- Your indigestion, gas and bloating issues will begin to resolve almost right away. This is because these real, whole and nutritious foods are irritant-free and will begin to allow your leaky gut syndrome to heal. As inflammatory particles no longer enter your bloodstream, your body starts to call off the autoimmune war it's been waging against itself.

- The simple act of removing gluten from your diet instantly begins to repair the damage of an inflamed brain. The blood brain barrier regains its impermeability and you start to see a reduction in mood swings, anxiety and depression. You may feel like "a weight has been lifted" from your mind and that your memory improves.

- Surprisingly, rheumatoid arthritis sufferers have reported improvement in pain and other autoimmune sufferers also see dramatic pain reduction, even in just 7 days. This is due to the fact that your food is no longer fueling inflammatory, ache-causing cytokines.

But don't take my word, or even years of research, for it! Start eating in the ancient, time-honored way that human beings were *designed* to eat and watch these amazing benefits multiply! Next, how you can make Paleo an inflammation-banishing lifestyle that heals you continually!

Chapter 10

An Anti-Inflammatory Lifestyle to Keep the Burn Away Forever

When we started this journey together, it was very important to me that you knew this wasn't just another "diet" book. That's because no matter how fantastic a diet or way of eating is, it will never be enough to completely eradicate something as serious and pervasive as chronic inflammation. The truth is that the war against the raging flames can never be truly won unless you make some lifestyle adjustments. Don't worry, this isn't where I introduce you to an excruciating exercise routine or tell you that you have to take hundreds of supplements and vitamins. No, this is where I tell you that to deeply heal every burnt-out cell in your body, all you have to do is respect your body's natural instincts. At this point, you've already gotten a chance to experience the intense flame-quenching effects of switching to an anti-inflammatory way of eating. Now, try these anti-inflammatory ways of *being* to deal the final blow to chronic inflammation and enjoy all of the benefits your body richly deserves:

Vitamin D: This may come as a surprise to you but did you know that staying out of the sun can get you burned? I'm not talking about sunburn here. Instead, I mean the dangerous low-grade fever type of burn that comes from being constantly inflamed. Vitamin D may be the missing and vital link in your anti-inflammatory strategy. Here's what to do if you suspect you're not getting enough:

Simply step outside and bask in direct sunlight for a minimum of 15 minutes or until your skin turns its lightest shade of pink. At this point your body has just produced its daily dose of vitamin D3 (Cholecalciferol). If for any reason, you can't tolerate direct sunlight (certain autoimmune disorders increase sun intolerance), you can increase your intake of vitamin D rich wild-caught fatty fish such as mackerel, tuna, or salmon. Sardines are also an excellent source, as are egg yolks from free-range chickens.

Exercise: It's very important to strike the right balance here because while moderate to moderately high levels of physical activity are great anti-inflammatory weapons, if you're hitting the gym or pounding the track too hard, you're actually causing dangerous oxidation and inflammation.

Moderate exercises like long and brisk walks have been shown to effectively lower the levels of your body's inflammatory markers C-reactive protein but surprisingly, overdoing it can cause levels of CRP to rise. Our ancient ancestors never "exercised". Instead, they did daily tasks that required them to move their bodies in sustained but moderate ways. I recommend walking as the best possible option as you begin your anti-inflammatory process and afterwards, if you feel you can handle it, you can move in to slightly more strenuous forms of activity.

Stress Reduction: While it's not realistic to think that you can completely emulate the lower-stress lifestyles of ancient populations, there are still many beneficial ways to deal with the increased stressors of modern life. Why is stress such an issue? When it comes to inflammation-reduction, lowering your levels of chronic stress may be one of the most important firefighting tools you have. Stress has been shown to increase levels of pain, tissue and even organ damage in inflamed patients who suffer from autoimmune diseases like lupus, multiple sclerosis and diabetes. Levels of the inflammatory marker IL-6 skyrocket when stress is present. So what can you do to get rid of your inflammation-fueling stress?

Slow down, even if it's only for a moment. In the fast-paced race of modern life, if you can grab a minute to stop, take a deep breath or a short walk in the sun, you can literally send stress and inflammation levels plummeting.

In Blue Zones, the long-living inhabitants spend time connecting with friends and family. This has a heart-protective and inflammation-busting effect that rivals medications. The truth is that human beings are social animals, and feelings of loneliness or isolation can directly impact your health. Talking with those close to you about your challenges can help you deal with them in a more effective and less emotional way, meaning that you don't have to suffer from the anxiety and sadness that often comes along with excessive stress.

Sleep: "I'll sleep when I'm dead." How many times have you said that sentence without realizing that every night of poor or inadequate sleep brings deadly inflammation and disease into your life? Not getting enough sleep directly leads to sharp spikes in inflammatory markers, and has been linked to heart disease and strokes, even in young or otherwise healthy subjects. Getting less than 6 hours of sleep a night leads to high inflammatory markers, including fibrinogen, IL-6 and CRP. This is important because raised inflammatory markers mean that you are 3 times more likely to have a fatal heart attack than the average person. Our ancestors rose with the sun rise and slept when the sun went down, giving themselves plenty of time to repair any physical damage. An added benefit of getting 8 or more hours of sleep is decreased pain and even abdominal weight loss so make sure you're giving your body the healing rewards of deep sleep.

Powerful Anti-Inflammatory Spices: Add these potent firefighting spices to your diet for a final anti-inflammatory step that's sure to give you lasting rejuvenation and relief:

Turmeric: If you're suffering from inflammatory arthritis or other autoimmune disorders, turmeric may be the most effective anti-inflammation treatment out there. This bright yellow root has been shown to give people inflammation-relief that rivals even the strongest painkillers and because it is natural, it provides this healing without any of the negative side effects of toxic drugs. Avoid taking turmeric supplements in pill form as this is far from being the purest or most natural form of turmeric. Instead, use this amazing anti-inflammatory as it's been consumed for centuries, ground and taken with water or mixed into meals. This one action will speed up your healing and revitalize everything from your joints to your brain cells!

Ginger: Ginger's amazing anti-inflammatory properties have been vaunted for over 2000 years in ancient populations around the globe. With the modern epidemic of inflammatory disease, this punchy spice can deliver a knockout blow to inflammation's last traces so add it to your natural anti-inflammatory diet today. How does it work? Ginger is full of anti-inflammatory substances called gingerols that easily fight inflammation and even work to repair its after effects. Tests show that those with osteoarthritis that is resistant to pain medication experience significant relief from pain and swelling when taking ginger.

Cayenne: Cayenne contains ample amounts of super anti-inflammatory substances capsaicinoids. With a proven track record in relieving everything from indigestion and supporting weight loss to banishing inflammation-led migraines and arthritic joint pain, this spice can literally change your life!

The Takeaway: Now that you've been introduced to the supreme inflammation firefighters and have been following the steps required to get you feeling, looking and living at your ultimate level, I'll share one last top tip with you to get you through the first weeks and then months of your brand new healing, revitalizing life: Perseverance. You can't buy it in stores but it really will be that final paramount ingredient to take your anti-inflammation battle to absolute victory. The results you should be seeing by now are sure to help you stay on track but if you ever waver and need a little encouragement, just take a look at the list of unbelievable benefits you've already started to prepare your body and mind to receive:

A slimmer, fitter, stronger you

- Ramped up energy levels

- An end to chronic fatigue

- Drastically reduced or completely eliminated pains, aches and swelling

- Improved mood

- Reduction in depression /anxiety

- Real sense of well-being

- Reduced bloating

- Visible weight loss that is easy to keep off

- A youthful, healthy complexion

- Great muscle tone

- Dramatically reduced risk of major killers like diabetes, heart disease and cancer

- A healed pancreas and normalized insulin secretion

- Reduction in cholesterol levels

- No more leaky gut syndrome

- An end to seasonal allergies

- Deep restful sleep

- An end to leaky brain syndrome

- Improved focus and concentration

- Enhanced productivity and creativity

- Boosted memory

- Mental clarity

Take a moment to let that soak in and applaud yourself for making the bold, brave moves that have brought you closer to complete healing and an optimal life. In the days ahead, if you find yourself confused about which choices to make, refer back to this book and let it be your guide. When you feel those familiar pangs or aches, don't hesitate to reach for these pages and call in those elite firefighters that are guaranteed to rescue you from the burn and beat out those flames.

As long as you keep making decisions that honor your body's processes, the wildfire of inflammation will stay gone for good. Remember that the anti-inflammatory guide you've received here is not another strict and joyless diet. With intensely flavorful and nourishing food options, exercise that comes naturally and time set aside to unwind and restore, you will be able to fully enjoy the vibrant, pain-free life you've always dreamed of! I wish you the very best of rejuvenation and health as you continue on your life-changing journey!

Are you ready to start some of that enjoyment right away? Turn to the recipe index for tantalizing anti-inflammatory recipes so good, you'll wonder why you didn't always eat this way!

Recipe Index

Delicious anti-inflammatory meals to get you started on your brand new, burn-free, slimmed – down and vibrant life! Enjoy them in good health!

Breakfast Recipes

Honey Apple Nut Paleo Granola

Almonds, walnuts & cashews offer an anti-inflammatory boost first thing in the morning.

Serves: Makes about 1 weeks' worth of breakfast granola, store in airtight container.

Ingredients

- 3 cups untoasted almonds

- 1 cup untoasted walnuts

- 1 cup untoasted cashew

- 2 cups dried apple slices

- 2 cups untoasted pumpkin seeds

- ½ cups dried cranberries

- ½ cup of pure coconut oil

- 1/3 cup honey

- 1 teaspoon ground cinnamon

- ½ teaspoon of pure vanilla seed powder

- ½ teaspoon kosher salt

Cooking Instructions:

1. Preheat your oven to 275-300 degrees F.

2. Mix all ingredients together thoroughly in a large mixing bowl.

3. Pour your mix out onto a baking sheet pre-oiled with coconut oil.

4. Allow to bake for 30 minutes, being careful not to let it burn.

5. Make sure your finished granola cools before you serve it.

Blood-Purifying Beet and Lemon Juice:

This juice uses the blood cleansing powers of beet and the diuretic effect of lemon to effectively pull out any remnants of your former sugar, simple carb, gluten and additives filled eating habits, setting the stage for the healing to begin.

Serves: 2

Ingredients:

- 1 ½ large beets, peeled and quartered
- The juice of 1 whole lemon
- ½ teaspoon of ground ginger

Instructions:

Put all ingredients through juicer. Serve immediately to preserve freshness.

Inflammation Quenching Spinach and Apple Juice: This juice employs the alpha-linoleic acid (ALA) found in spinach, a substance that reduces a wide range of inflammatory cytokines by over 40% and the quercetin found in apples.

Serves: 2

Ingredients

- 4 apples, cored
- 2 cups spinach

Instructions:

Cut items into suitable size and juice. Serve immediately to preserve freshness.

Burn-Busting Broccoli, Cherry and Blueberry Smoothie: Studies have shown the efficacy of sulforaphane, a substance found in broccoli, in halting inflammatory and destructive enzymes. Broccoli has been found to be particularly helpful in fending off the searing joint pain of rheumatoid arthritis so this is a great choice if you're suffering from similar autoimmune aches. Choose cherries for their ability to soothe chronically inflamed blood vessels and blueberries for their protective and rejuvenating effects on the brain and nervous system.

Serves: 3 to 4

Ingredients:

- 1 large head of broccoli
- 1 cup pitted cherries
- 1 cup blueberries
- ½ cup coconut milk

Instructions:

Blend all ingredients together and serve immediately to preserve freshness.

Paleo Treat Pancakes

These pancakes make for an excellent occasional treat that will help ward off grain-cravings. Free-range eggs are full of anti-inflammatory omega-3 and ground ginger and cinnamon add a dash of anti-swelling power.

Serves: 2

- **Ingredients:**
- 3 medium ripe bananas
- 2 large free-range eggs
- 1/3 cup of cashew butter
- ½ teaspoon ground ginger

- Dash of cinnamon

- Dash of nutmeg

Instructions:

Mix all ingredients well in a food processor

Oil your preheated pan with either olive oil or coconut oil

Pour batter onto pan in small amounts, allowing each pancake to cook about 4 minutes on each side

Serve warm for best results

Lunch & Dinner Recipes

Avocado Beef Cups on a Bed of Spinach

Avocados are extremely anti-inflammatory and soothe a leaky gut while grass-fed, pastured beef contains flame fighting omega-3. Garlic is a powerful swelling reducer and blood sugar regulator while spinach contains known anti-inflammatory compounds in its phytonutrients.

Serves: 2-3

Ingredients:

- 4 medium avocadoes
- 6 oz. of grass-fed, pastured ground beef
- 5 cups fresh spinach leaves
- 1 medium onion finely diced
- 4 cloves of garlic finely diced
- 1 tablespoon extra-virgin olive oil
- 1½ teaspoon turmeric
- 1 large lemon

Instructions:

Open all 4 avocadoes lengthwise, turning them into little serving cups and squeeze lemon onto them

In a skillet, combine olive oil, ground beef, onion, garlic and turmeric until lightly browned

Arrange spinach on serving platter and place avocados on it

Fill avocado cups with ground beef mixture, allowing skillet juices to season the spinach leaves.

Serve warm or room temperature, as desired

Sardine and Mushroom Tossed Salad

Sardines are absolutely chockfull of omega-3, providing a burn-beating blast without the risk of mercury, garlic and onions both have anti-swelling properties that can help with rheumatoid arthritis, lupus or other autoimmune disorder and mushrooms provide filling, low-calorie satisfaction.

Serves: 3-4

Ingredients:

- ½ cup sardines
- 4 cups fresh lettuce
- ½ cup fresh mushrooms
- 2 red onions chopped
- 10 cloves minced garlic
- Juice from 1 ½ limes
- 5 tablespoons olive oil

Instructions:

In a small bowl whisk together olive oil, garlic, lime juice and set aside

In a large salad bowl, combine lettuce, sardines, mushrooms and onions

Pour dressing in small bowl over salad and serve.

Spiralizer Spinach Carrot Pasta (A Paleo & Vegan Meal)

Carrots are loaded with anti-oxidants while spinach's phytonutrients ease inflammatory responses. Turmeric contributes to pain-relief.

Serves: 3

Ingredients:

- 3 large carrots made into noodles with a spiralizer or thinly sliced by hand

- Creamy white pasta sauce:

- 1 large diced yellow onion

- ½ cup mushrooms

- ½ cup almond milk

- ½ teaspoon turmeric

- 10 cloves of garlic minced

- ½ cup spinach

- Dash nutmeg

- 4 large tablespoons extra-virgin olive oil

- 1 tablespoon raw, grass-fed butter to serve

Instructions:

Use a spiralizer on your carrots and set aside. In a sauce pan slightly blanch spinach leaves. In a separate saucepan, brown onions in olive oil until golden and add mushrooms, garlic, turmeric, nutmeg and almond milk. Add spinach and allow mixture to thicken. Pour over bowl of carrot pasta and serve warm with a dollop of raw, grass-fed butter.

Kimchi, Grilled Beets and Beef Sliders

The fermented power of kimchi's probiotics provides a huge anti-pain boost for those suffering autoimmune disorders while beets purify the blood and beef offers a dose of joint, tissue and organ soothing omega-3.

Serves: 2

Ingredients:

- 3 large beets, sliced into discs

- 1 large red onion

- ¼ cup kimchi

- 6 oz. grass-fed pastured ground beef

- 1 large avocado

- 5 tablespoons live yogurt

Instructions:

Slice the beets into discs and place on grill

Form beef into patties and also grill

Slice large onion and place on grill

In a bowl combine, mashed avocado, live yogurt and kimchi to make a sauce

Remove items from grill and layer starting with beets, then beef patties on beets, kimchi avocado yogurt sauce on patties and finally top with grilled onions. Enjoy warm.

Paleo Kale Chips

These veggie chips make a great snack alternative to toxic, packaged chips. Kale is a fantastic source of nutrition, packing in vitamin C, E, & K while the garlic and herbs allow for improved circulation, reducing inflammation.

Serves: 3

Ingredients:

- Large bunch of kale
- 1 teaspoon minced garlic
- 4 tablespoons animal fat

- Salt and oregano/parsley (or other seasoning as desired)

Instructions:

Cut kale to chip shape and size

Mix them with animal fat

Season them with salt and oregano/parsley

Bake evenly in pre-heated oven for 25 minutes

Remove, sprinkle with minced garlic, allow to cool and serve.

Baked Wild Salmon on a Bed of Asparagus

Wild-caught salmon is one of the best sources of inflammation-banishing omega-3 available. Asparagus is a well-known blood-detoxifier and substituting asparagus for the more traditional heavy carb staples also provides a low-glycemic meal that works perfectly as a blood-sugar stabilizing dinner.

Serves: 4

Ingredients:

- 25 oz. of wild-caught salmon
- 1 bunch of asparagus spears
- 2 teaspoons dill
- Juice from 1 large lemon
- 4 tablespoons extra-virgin olive oil

Instructions:

Combine lemon juice and olive oil in a small bowl

Steam asparagus spears in salted water until tender.

Top salmon with dill and bake in oven for 30 minutes at 375 degrees F, keeping an eye on it throughout.

Serve salmon on a bed of asparagus and drizzle with lemon, olive oil dressing

<u>Paleo Desserts</u>- Paleo Desserts are very simple to make and can be prepared in a rush, warding off those sugar emergencies. What you won't get: Sugar, high fructose corn syrup, additives, gluten or grains. What you will get:

Whole, real, inflammation-fighting goodness that tastes better than you could ever imagine!

Simply Sweet Paleo Pineapple

This ultra-simple dessert is a quick, truly easy paleo sweet to help take the edge off of dessert cravings. Pineapples contain high levels of bromelain, a natural and intense anti-inflammatory that works wonders on everything from gout to arthritis. Enjoy this dessert for a pain and swelling- busting nightcap.

Serves: 5-6

Ingredients:

- 1 large whole pineapple
- 1 tablespoon coconut oil

- Juice from 1 ½ large limes
- Dash of sea salt

Instructions:

Remove rough exterior of pineapple and slice into circular discs

Heat a pan and swirl with coconut oil

Place discs of pineapple down on hot pan, allowing them to sear slightly on one side before flipping

Drench with lime juice, sprinkle with sea salt and enjoy!

Strawberry Mango Freeze

Strawberries and mangoes are packed with damage repairing antioxidants while mint is well-known both for its swelling-reducing powers and its ability to promote sharper thinking, combatting inflammatory damage in your most important organ.

Serves: 3

Ingredients:

- 1 cup frozen strawberries
- 1 cup cubed frozen mango
- 2 cups creamy almond milk, chilled
- 1 lime
- Sprigs of fresh mint

Instructions:

In a blender, blend strawberries, mango cubes, mint and almond milk until creamy.

Pour mixture into separate dessert glasses and allow to chill in freezer until semi-frozen.

Serve doused in lime juice.

Chocolate Dipped Medjool Dates

Medjool dates are the perfect, rare, pick-me-up when sugar is on your mind. Their natural sweetness sends cravings running but do be careful about eating these close to bedtime. As an added bonus, they have magnesium which allows for optimal vitamin D absorption. Note: Their high-glycemic index score means that they should be eaten earlier in the day, when you'll have time to combat their blood-glucose raising effects.

Serves: 3

Ingredients:

- 20 large, pit-free Medjool dates at room temperature
- Pure organic dark chocolate bar (gluten, grain, additives, sugar-free)
- Tooth picks

Instructions:

Melt the organic dark chocolate in a small sauce pan

Spear the Medjool dates with toothpicks

Dip each date in the warm, melted chocolate and serve on a platter

Other books by author

50 Foods to avoid to lose weight and stay

Happy and Healthy